THE MEDICAID HANDBOOK

A User's Guide to Florida Medicaid

Authors

Joseph F. Pippen, Jr., J.D.
&
John R. Frazier J.D., LL.M.

Published by
PEARTREE®
P.O. Box 14533
Clearwater, Florida 33766-4533

Printed in the United States of America

Book Order Department
727-586-3306

10 9 8 7 6 5 4 3 2 1

CIP
Pippen, Joseph F. Jr. 1947
  The Medicaid handbook: a user's guide to Florida medicaid / Joseph F. Pippen, Jr.,
  John R. Frazier
    p. cm
  ISBN 0935343-64-4
  1.Medicaid--Florida--Handbooks, manuals, etc. 2. Medicaid--Handbooks, manuals, etc.
I. Frazier, John R., 1963- II. Title.

  RA412.45.F6P57 2005
  368.4'2009759--dc22   LC 2005056562

Disclaimer: This book is intended to answer the most often asked questions concerning legal
issues. This book is not intended as a substitute for legal counsel and questions will be answered
in general context. Specific legal questions usually have too many variables to give concise, legal
answers covering all ramifications. Please consult your own attorney for recent changes in the
law.

ABOUT THE AUTHOR

Joseph F. Pippen, Jr. J.D.

JOSEPH FRANKLIN PIPPEN, JR.- Attorney, was born in 1947 in Richmond, Virginia. He graduated from Virginia Tech in 1969 with a degree in economics. He also served in the National Guard as a captain of a combat engineering group. From 1969 until 1980, he was an executive in management positions in the fields of manufacturing, production control, marketing, purchasing, finance and public relations.

From 1980 through part of 1982, Joe Pippen served as general manager of Micro-Plate, Inc. of Florida and helped guide the small, high-tech company into becoming a major force in the printed circuit-board industry.

Joe Pippen graduated from the University of Baltimore Law School in 1975 with a Juris Doctorate and has been practicing law since 1982. His law firm has grown to offices in Largo, Sun City Center, Tampa, Zephyrhills, Live Oak, Haines City, Lakeland and Bradenton. His law firm consists of eight attorneys that practice in the areas of estate and tax planning, real estate, Medicaid and family law issues. He has also taught Business Law and Management at Anne Arundel Community College and at St. Petersburg College.

Besides his noteworthy business and career accomplishments, Pippen has numerous other achievements to his credit. He has been honored four times as one of the "Outstanding Men of America," has been listed in Who's Who in Finance and Industry and Who's Who in American Law. He also has been cited as one of the "Outstanding Volunteer Activists." Of all his achievements, Pippen is most proud of the millions of dollars he has raised for the United Way and his volunteer role with young people and the free enterprise system through the Hugh O'Brien Youth Foundation.

Pippen is a noted speaker and lecturer on motivational and personal dynamic subjects as well as management and legal topics. His weekly column, "Ask an Attorney," appeared in several local newspapers, and he has hosted a continuous weekly radio call-in show entitled "Ask an Attorney" since 1985. He also has hosted a national radio call-in show with the same title on the Sun Radio Network.

He is married to his high-school sweetheart, Beverly, and they have two sons, Trey and Troy, and two grandsons, Austin and Trevor. They presently reside in Largo, Florida.

ABOUT THE AUTHOR

John Richard Frazier, J.D., LL.M.

John Richard Frazier was born in 1962 in Jersey City, New Jersey. He Graduated Cum Laude from Hampden-Sydney College in Virginia with a B.A. in Economics in 1986. He received his Master's degree in Business Administration from Virginia Tech in 1994; graduated Cum Laude from the University of Toledo, College of Law in 1997; and received his LL.M. in Taxation from the University of Florida, College of Law in 1998.

He is licensed to practice Law in both Florida and Georgia, and he practices primarily in the fields of Elder Law, Estate Planning, Asset Protection, Taxation, Medicaid Planning and Business Organizations.

He is also a member of the National Academy of Elder Law Attorneys of Florida Elder Law Attorneys, and the Florida Bar Elder Law Section.

A special thanks to Patrick Smith, Law student at North Carolina Law School, who provided research and much assistance in preparing this information.

Please be advised that MEDICAID Laws are revised every January and July.

Please consult an Elder Law Attorney for recent changes.

Medicaid rules change periodically

Refer to web site at
http://www. Attypip.com

TABLE OF CONTENTS

THE MEDICAID HANDBOOK

III. Medicaid Planning 21

IV. Medicaid Quick Reference Guide 40

Chapter I
MEDICAID
BACKGROUND INFORMATION

Medicaid History

Medicaid began in the 1960's as a welfare program designed to provide medical assistance to the impoverished. As a result of this policy, many elderly couples who could not afford to pay for the cost of a nursing home were forced to impoverish themselves in order to qualify for Medicaid. Fortunately, Congress responded to this tragic consequence.

The Medicare Catastrophic Coverage Act of 1988 provided relief from self-impoverishment by allowing those seeking to qualify for Medicaid to keep certain assets and income so long as the assets and income did not rise above certain levels. This reform transformed the nature of Medicaid from a welfare program for the impoverished to a general medical insurance program for those who met the need, asset, and income requirements.

Medicaid reform continued in 1996 when Congress made it illegal for anyone to transfer assets in order to qualify for Medicaid. Nevertheless, Congress amended this law in 1997 to allow persons to transfer assets to qualify for Medicaid but made it illegal for anyone to charge a fee for advice or counseling on how to transfer such assets in order to qualify for Medicaid. Ultimately, in 1998 the Attorney General declared that the law limiting advice and counseling would not be enforced since it violated the First Amendment's protection of freedom of speech. Subsequent court cases have supported the Attorney General's decision.

Thus, attorneys may provide Medicaid Planning in order to protect the assets of clients who are seeking to qualify for Medicaid coverage. Indeed, many attorneys now specialize in Medicaid Planning. Medicaid planning involves a series of strategies that are designed to assist a person in qualifying for Medicaid.

Medicaid Coverage

Q: What does Medicaid cover?

A: Medicaid covers the cost of nursing home care, in-patient and out-patient medical care, surgery, hospitalization, transportation to and from the hospital, dialysis, psychiatric care and counseling, medical supplies, and medication. Medicaid does <u>not</u> cover hearing aids, eyeglasses, or dental care.

Q: Does Medicaid pay for the cost of an Assisted Living Facility (ALF) ?

A: Yes. Medicaid does cover the cost of an ALF for persons who qualify for Medicaid. However, the funding available to cover the cost of an ALF is limited.

Q: Is Medicaid available only to the elderly?

A: In the state of Florida, Medicaid may be available to low income families with children, elderly persons, disabled persons, pregnant women, children, and some non-citizens.

4

Medicaid vs. Medicare

Q: What are the differences between Medicare and Medicaid?

A: There are several key differences between Medicare and Medicaid. Medicare is a federally run health insurance program for seniors who contributed to Medicare. Medicaid is a partnership between the state and federal governments that provides medical assistance to those who meet certain need, income, and asset requirements. Furthermore, while Medicare requirements are uniform throughout the United States, Medicaid requirements vary from state to state. Thus, it is important to consult with an Elder Law attorney in your state regarding your Medicaid eligibility.

Example: George Jones is 85 years old and has been in the hospital for five days following a stroke and injuries suffered from a fall after the stroke. His doctor has advised the family that George will need long term care in a nursing home. Upon admission to a facility which is licensed to accept both Medicare and Medicaid, George is eligible for the following: George <u>may</u> be eligible for 20 days of full coverage in the nursing home under Medicare. George <u>may</u> be eligible for partial coverage under Medicare for 21-100 days, with a deductible of $119.00 per day. In order to obtain coverage under Medicaid, George must meet the three-part test for Medicaid eligibility.

Florida Department of Children and Families

Q: What is the Florida Department of Children and Families?

A: The Department of Children and Families is the state government agency that determines an applicant's eligibility for Medicaid.

Medicaid Institutional Care Program

Q: What is the Medicaid Institutional Care Program?

A: The Medicaid Institutional Care Program (ICP) is operated by the state and federal governments and provides assistance for nursing home costs to those individuals who qualify. Because of the increase in the cost of nursing home care, the ICP is one of the most popular Medicaid programs.

Florida Department of Elder Affairs C.A.R.E.S. Unit

Q: What is the Florida Department of Elder Affairs C.A.R.E.S. Unit?

A: C.A.R.E.S. stands for Comprehensive, Assessment, Review and Evaluation Services. C.A.R.E.S. is a federally mandated program that assesses a Medicaid applicant's needs and required level of care for nursing home and assisted living Medicaid programs.

Medicaid Waiver Programs

Q: What are the Medicaid Waiver Programs?

A: Medicaid Waiver Programs provide a variety of home and community based services to those who are at risk of being admitted to a nursing home. Medicaid funds pay for these programs. Each participant in a Medicaid Waiver Program is assigned a caseworker who works to see that the participant's needs are met.

Long Term Care Diversion Program

Q: What is the Long Term Care Diversion Program?

A: The Long Term Care Diversion Program is a Medicaid Waiver Program that provides services, such as preventative health care and prescription drugs to the elderly while allowing them to remain at home. However, the funding for this program is limited.

Chapter II
MEDICAID ELIGIBILITY REQUIREMENTS

Basic Eligibility Requirements

Q: What are the basic requirements for a person to be eligible for Medicaid coverage of the cost of nursing home care?

A: There is a three-pronged test that an applicant must pass in order to be eligible for Medicaid coverage of nursing home costs. The three prongs are: 1) a medical needs-based test, 2) an assets test, and 3) an income test. Each of these tests is discussed in detail in the subsequent sections of this handbook. Nevertheless, do not be alarmed if, after reading the descriptions of the requirements, you find yourself to have exceeded the limits for Medicaid eligibility. Medicaid planning can help. In fact, often times, after proper Medicaid planning those who thought themselves ineligible for Medicaid are actually found to be eligible for Medicaid coverage of their nursing home costs.

Needs-Based Test

Q: What are the Needs-Based Standards for Medicaid eligibility?

A: To meet the Needs-Based Standard for Medicaid Eligibility an individual must be aged 65 or older or disabled.

Example: Jane Smith is 78 years old and suffers from Chronic Obstructive Pulmonary Disease (COPD) and Alzheimer's disorder. She is no longer able to live independently or care for herself. She has recently been discharged from an assisted living facility due to her having become a serious fall risk. Jane will meet the medically necessary level of care needed to qualify for Medicaid.

Asset Test

Q: What is the Resource Allowance for an Individual (Assets Test)?

A: This term describes the maximum asset

allowance that a Medicaid applicant may keep and still maintain Medicaid eligibility. Note that there are exempt assets that a Medicaid applicant may retain without having such assets included in the resource allowance calculation. Exempt assets include: 1) homestead property or personal residence, 2) one automobile, 3) certain specially structured contracts and some promissory notes, 4) household furnishings, 5) one burial savings account (under $2,500.00) per spouse, 6) some life insurance contracts, 7) household items and most personal effects, and 8) $99,540.00 in any type of assets for the nursing home patient's community spouse. In the state of Florida for the year 2006, the resource allowance for an individual is $2,000.00

Example: Diana Folwell owns her own mobile home, one car, clothing, furniture, and personal effects. She has one checking account with $800.00 in it, a group life insurance policy, and a cremation contract for which she paid $1,500.00. Diana will meet the $2,000.00 asset test for a single person.

Q: What is the Resource Allowance for a Couple (both husband and wife) in a nursing home?

A: This term describes the maximum asset allowance that a husband and wife may maintain if both husband and wife are Medicaid applicants living in a nursing home. The resource allowance, for the year 2006 for a couple who lives in the state of Florida, is $3,000.00.

Minimum Monthly Maintenance Needs Allowance

Q: What is the Minimum Monthly Maintenance Needs Allowance?

A: This term describes the minimum allowable income that the state must protect for the spouse of an institutionalized person who is seeking Medicaid coverage. This amount is not included in determining the Medicaid applicant's eligibility. In the state of Florida for the year 2006, the minimum monthly maintenance needs allowance is $1,604.00.

Example: Jane Smith receives $500.00 per month in social security and her husband, Jim Smith, who is on Medicaid in a nursing home, receives $1,000.00 per month in social security. This is the only income either receives. Jane Smith will be able to keep all of her husband's social security because the combined total income between Jane and Jim Smith is less than $1,604.00. There will be no cost for the nursing home in this situation.

Maximum Monthly Maintenance Needs Allowance

Q: What is the Maximum Monthly Maintenance Needs Allowance?

A: This term describes the maximum asset allowance that the state will protect for the spouse of an institutionalized person who is seeking Medicaid coverage. Some states have chosen to combine the maximum and minimum monthly maintenance needs allowances into a single figure. However, the state of Florida maintains two separate figures for the maximum and minimum amounts. In the state of Florida for the year 2006, the maximum monthly maintenance needs allowance is $2,489.00

Example: Jane Smith receives $2,500.00 per month in gross social security and pension, and Jim Smith, her husband and a nursing home patient, receives only $500.00 per month in gross social security. Jane will not be entitled to any of her husband's income, and the cost of the nursing home will be $465.00 per month ($500.00 - $35.00 personal needs allowance).

Community Spouse Resource Allowance

Q: What is the Community Spouse Resource Allowance?

A: This term describes the maximum amount of resources that a non-institutionalized spouse of an institutionalized Medicaid applicant may maintain. For the state of Florida for the year 2006, the community spouse resource allowance is $99,540.00.

Example: Jane and Jim Smith own a home worth $100,000.00, one car, clothing, furniture, $50,000.00 in bank accounts, and each owns one term-life insurance policy with no cash value. If Jim goes into a nursing home and Jane stays at home, Jane will be below the $99,540.00 community spouse resource allowance.

Monthly Personal Needs Allowance

Q: What is the Monthly Personal Needs Allowance?

A: This term describes the amount that the state permits a Medicaid applicant to retain for personal needs. In the state of Florida for the year 2006, the monthly personal needs allowance is $35.00.

Example: Tom Smith is a single person on Medicaid in a nursing home. His gross income is $1,000.00 per month. Tom is allowed to keep $35.00 of his income for his personal use. The cost of the nursing home is $965.00 per month.

Income Test

Q: What is the Income Cap Amount (Institutional Care Program Income/Long Term Care Diversion Program)?

A: This term describes the maximum amount of gross income that a Medicaid applicant may have and still be eligible for Medicaid coverage of the cost of a nursing home. Note that this term describes a cap on "gross" income. Thus, Medicare Part B premiums, insurance premiums, tax deductions, as well as other deductions, must be added to the applicant's income in determining whether the applicant is under the income cap amount. The income cap is strictly enforced. A Medicaid applicant who is over the income cap by even $1 will be ineligible for Medicaid even though they have met the other tests for eligibility. However, there is no limit on the level of income of the Medicaid applicant's spouse. In the state of Florida for the year 2006, the income cap amount is $1,809.00 per month.

Example: Steve Smith receives $2,000.00 per month in gross social security and pension. The current income cap in Florida is

$1,809.00 per month in gross income. In order to qualify for Medicaid, Steve will have to establish, and properly fund each month, an Irrevocable Income-Only Trust.

Shelter Standard

Q: What is the Shelter Standard?

A: Once a community spouse's shelter cost rises above the shelter standard, the community spouse may collect income from the institutionalized spouse for the cost of shelter. The current Florida shelter standard is $482.00. When the cost of shelter exceeds the shelter standard the minimum monthly needs allowance may be increased to meet the shelter costs up to the maximum monthly maintenance needs allowance.

Example: Jane Smith receives $1,600.00 per month in gross social security, and her husband Tom Smith receives $2,000.00 per month in gross social security and pension. If Jane Smith's shelter expenses (i.e., mortgage payment, monthly condo maintenance fee, electric bill, water bill, sewage bill, property tax bill, and property insurance bill) exceed $482.00 per month, Jane will be entitled to some of her husband's income each month. Tom is in a nursing home on Medicaid.

Medicaid Eligibility for Non-U.S. Citizens

Q: What are the Medicaid Qualifications for Non-U.S. citizens?

A: Generally, a person that is not a U.S. citizen is not eligible for Medicaid coverage. However, a non-resident alien who has been in the country for 5 years or longer is eligible for Medicaid coverage.

Example: Alex Smith is a Canadian citizen who has resided in the United States for only two years. Alex does not meet the eligibility residency requirement to become qualified for Medicaid.

Medicaid Requirements in Different States

Q: Are the Medicaid requirements the same throughout the different states?

A: No. Different states have different requirements for Medicaid eligibility. Therefore, it is important that you consult with an Elder Law attorney in your state regarding the specific eligibility requirements for Medicaid in that state. Florida's asset protection laws are some of the most generous in the country. Under Florida Statute §222, homesteads, retirement accounts, IRAs, annuities, and $1,000.00 of personal property items are protected from creditors.

Chapter III
MEDICAID PLANNING

Medicaid Planning

Q: What is Medicaid Planning?

A: Medicaid Planning provides Medicaid applicants with assistance in understanding the complex nature of the Medicaid application process. Proper Medicaid Planning can help Medicaid applicants avoid the pitfalls of Medicaid law, maximize their asset protection, and ultimately gain Medicaid benefits.

Transfer of Assets

Q: Can a person transfer less than $12,000.00 a year to a person, thereby avoiding gift taxation, without reporting such transfer during the Medicaid application process?

A: Avoidance of the gift tax does not determine whether a transfer must be reported during the Medicaid application process. If the transfer occurs within the applicable look-back period for the transfer, then the transfer must be reported. However, it is important to note that not all transfers made within the look back period disqualify a person for Medicaid eligibility.

Q: Should a Medicaid applicant transfer all or most of his assets to another person or trust prior to his Medicaid application?

A: No. Oftentimes, such transfers are within the 36 month look-back period for transfers to individuals or within the 60 month look-back period for transfers to irrevocable trusts and, therefore, may potentially create a period of ineligibility for the Medicaid applicant. The most prudent strategy is to consult with a Medicaid Planning attorney *prior* to any transfers.

Q: Is it illegal to transfer assets in order to qualify for Medicaid?

A: After the 1996 Kennedy-Kassebaum Health

Care Bill, it was illegal to transfer assets in order to qualify for Medicaid. However, this provision was repealed in 1997 and replaced with a law that made it illegal to charge someone for counseling on how to transfer assets to qualify for Medicaid. Nevertheless, in 1998 the Attorney General declared that this law would not be enforced since it violated the First Amendment's protection of free speech.

Look-Back Periods

Q: What are the Look-Back Periods for determining Medicaid eligibility?

A: Look-back periods require that all transfers made during such periods be disclosed during the Medicaid application process. There are two look-back periods. For transfers made to an irrevocable trust, the look back period is 60 months from the date of application for Medicaid. For transfers made to individuals, the look-back period is 36 months from the date of application for Medicaid.

Example: Joe Smith gifted $15,000.00 to his son Jim Smith last month. Joe had a stroke this month and needs long term nursing care. Joe has created a disqualification period of four months, and Joe is now ineligible for Medicaid for that period of time, unless he is able to "cure" the gift. This means some or the entire gift must be returned to Joe. Joe must also file form 709 between January 1 and April 15 of the year following the gift.

Example: Kelly Smith gave all of her assets, including her house, car, and bank accounts, to her daughter Kim. The amount of the transfer was $200,000.00. Kelly has created a disqualification period of 60 months for Medicaid, unless Kelly is able to "cure" the gift.

Example: Joe Smith gave his daughter a $30,000.00 graduation present two years ago. If Joe applies for Medicaid within three years of the gift, Joe must disclose that gift. However, a $30,000.00 gift two years ago, although it must be disclosed, would not create a period of ineligibility two years after the gift.

Divestment Penalty Divisor

Q: What is the Divestment Penalty Divisor?

A: This term describes the figure that is calculated by the state based upon the average cost of one month of nursing home care. If a Medicaid applicant transfers assets for less than the fair market value of the assets, the amount of the transfer is divided by the divestment penalty divisor to determine the Medicaid applicant's period of ineligibility for Medicaid. However, transfers made between a husband and wife are not considered transfers for Medicaid eligibility purposes and are, therefore, not subject to the penalty described above. In the state of Florida for the year 2006, the divestment penalty divisor is $3,300.00.

Example: Joe Smith gifted $33,000.00 to his son Jeffrey this month. The divestment penalty divisor is $3,300.00. $33,000.00 divided by $3,300.00 is 10. This means that Joe is not eligible for Medicaid for 10 months following the $33,000.00 gift, unless Joe "cures" the gift.

Qualified Special Needs Trust

Q: What is a Qualified Special Needs Trust?

A: Qualified special needs trusts prepare for the death of a spouse of a Medicaid recipient. The state of Florida has, in the past, required that a Medicaid recipient elect to take their elective share from the estate of a deceased spouse. The qualified special needs trust operates to avoid this potentially disqualifying event. A will is created that contains a testamentary special needs trust for the surviving spouse who is a Medicaid recipient. The trust must receive at least 30% of the deceased spouse's estate so that the elective share statute requirements are satisfied. Since this 30% of the deceased spouse's estate goes into the qualified special needs trust upon the death of the spouse, the Medicaid recipient continues his or her Medicaid eligibility.

Example: Jason Jones was born with severe disabilities and has been classified as disabled under social security for most of his life. Under his parents' will, his parents created a Qualified Special Needs Trust to hold their assets upon their death in order to provide supplemental support for Jason during his lifetime. If the Trust is drafted properly, Jason will be able to maintain his benefits under social security, and he will also be able to qualify for Medicaid benefits.

Qualified Income Trust

Q: What is a Qualified Income Trust?

A: Should a Medicaid applicant exceed the monthly income level that is required in order to qualify for Medicaid, a qualified income trust must be created to capture the excess income. However, the qualified income trust must be properly drafted and properly funded for each month that a person needs Medicaid qualification.

Example: Joe Smith has $2,000.00 per month in gross income. In order to qualify for Medicaid benefits, Joe will need to set up a Qualified Income Trust. The Trust can be set up by Joe if he has capacity, by his guardian upon petition and consent by a court of jurisdiction, or by an attorney in fact with a properly drafted power of attorney.

Personal Service Contracts

Q: What is a Personal Service Contract?

A: A person seeking to apply for Medicaid coverage may enter into a personal services contract with another person. The personal services contract will provide that the Medicaid applicant is to receive services from the other person, often called the caregiver, in exchange for personal or real property that is approximately equal to the value of the services rendered. This transfer of property is not a potentially disqualifying gift since the property is given to the caregiver in exchange for the personal services rendered and is approximately equal to the value of the services.

Example: Jane Smith is a resident in a nursing home. She has $2,000.00 in a checking account, a mobile home, and a car. She is a single person. She has one daughter named Regina who is Jane's primary care giver. In the current month, she gives $3,200.00 as a gift to Regina, and her attorney drafts a Personal Services Contract payable to Regina for $15,300.00 which will constitute gross income to Regina. Jane is able to qualify for Medicaid in the current month because the $15,300.00 Personal Services Contract is classified as payment for future services and not as a gift.

Medicaid Qualifying Annuity

Q: What is a Medicaid Qualifying Annuity?

A: A Medicaid Qualifying Annuity is one of the many tools that may be utilized in qualifying a person for Medicaid eligibility. The annuity must be immediate, non-assignable, and non-transferable.

Example: Tom Smith is single, owns a condominium and a car, and has $140,000.00 in a checking account. Tom needs to obtain nursing home benefits this month. Tom has three children. Tom's Power of Attorney established a $138,500.00 Medicaid Qualifying balloon style, single premium, immediate annuity with a life insurance company that issues Medicaid Qualifying annuities. Tom is now immediately qualified for Medicaid. The annuity has a beneficiary provision in which Tom's three children are equal beneficiaries. Upon Tom's death, Tom's children will receive the funds held in the annuity.

Durable Power of Attorney

Q: What is a Durable Power of Attorney and how does it relate to Medicaid Planning?

A: A Durable Power of Attorney is a document executed by a person to give someone else, called the attorney-in-fact, power to make certain decisions on his or her behalf. Should Medicaid Planning become necessary for an incapacitated person, certain powers must be included in the durable power of attorney in order for the attorney-in-fact to be able to conduct such planning activities. Thus, it is important to have an attorney draft a durable power of attorney in order to insure that all the necessary powers are included.

"Lady Bird" Deeds

Q: What are "Lady Bird" Deeds?

A: "Lady Bird" Deeds transfer property through a beneficiary deed-like instrument. The Lady Bird Deed is utilized in Medicaid Planning because, though revocable by the grantor of the deed, it is a non-countable asset for Medicaid qualification.

Example: Jane Smith is a single individual who owns a condominium and a jointly held checking account. Jane needs to apply for Medicaid benefits and would like to avoid probate upon her death. Jane has one daughter who is the 100% beneficiary in Jane's will. Jane's attorney drafts a properly written life estate Lady Bird deed transferring a remainder interest in the condominium to her daughter upon Jane's death. The transfer of the remainder interest to the daughter under the Lady Bird deed does not create a disqualification period for Medicaid, whereas the standard Life Estate deed would have created a disqualification period.

Protection of Homestead

Q: Must a Medicaid applicant sell his or her home in order to gain Medicaid eligibility?

A: No. While a Medicaid applicant must meet asset requirements, along with need and income requirements in order to qualify for Medicaid, the applicant's home is an exempt asset and is not included in the determination of the applicant's asset level so long as the home is the person's homestead. Other exempt assets include a Medicaid applicant's car and an irrevocable burial contract.

Example: Tom Smith is a single individual who lives in a beach front condominium with a fair market value that has increased to 1.2 million dollars. Tom's only other asset is a checking account with $1,500.00 in it. Even though Tom's net worth is more than 1 million dollars, Tom is qualified for Medicaid because the condominium is a non-countable asset.

Private Pay

Q: Should a person use private pay to cover the cost of a nursing home instead of turning to Medicaid?

A: Most people that decide to use private pay to cover their own or a loved one's nursing home costs deplete their available assets within a couple of years. Thus, usually only the very wealthy are able to pay privately for the duration of their nursing home care. For those that cannot afford to pay privately for the entire duration of their nursing home care, they will, more than likely, apply for Medicaid. Planning for Medicaid will preserve your assets for family and loved ones and ease the burden that private pay places on a family's budget.

Example: Aunt Bessie has been in a nursing home for the past six years, at a cost of $200.00 per day. Not including the cost of medication and other incidental expenses, Bessie has spent $432,000.00 on the nursing home in the past six years.

Long Term Care Insurance

Q: Should a person use long term care insurance to pay for nursing home expenses?

A: The major benefit to long term care insurance is the fact that it often covers more than just the cost of a nursing home. However, the major downside to long term care insurance is the cost associated with such insurance. Additionally, individuals should also consider that if their long term care insurance is not sufficient to cover the entire cost of their nursing home care and they need to apply for Medicaid coverage, payments from their long term care insurance may count as income and push them over the income cap for Medicaid eligibility.

Example: Bob Jones purchased a long term care insurance policy 25 years ago which paid $80.00 per day for the cost of a nursing home. When Bob purchased the contract, the average cost of a nursing home was $80.00 per day. The policy has no provision for adjustments for inflation, so the policy will only pay $2,400.00 per month. Bob's nursing home costs $200.00 per day, so he will have an out-of-pocket expense of $3,600.00 per month if he does not become qualified for Medicaid.

Family Contribution

Q: Should family contribution be used to support an elderly loved one that requires long term care?

A: The primary advantage of family contribution for the care of a loved one is the satisfaction that the family derives from knowing that the family, as opposed to a non-family member, is caring for the loved one. However, there are several major disadvantages to family contribution for the long term care of a loved one. The first is the financial strain that such contribution places on the family. Oftentimes when a family contributes to cover the nursing home costs of a loved one, one or more family members are hindered from saving for their own retirement or for the higher education of younger family members. Furthermore, when a family contributes to the care of an elderly loved one, it often requires one or more family members to take time away from their jobs in order to provide care for the elderly family member, oftentimes adding to existing financial strain. Medicaid planning can provide the elderly family member with the long term care that he or she needs and can avoid the hardships posed by family contribution.

Medicaid Estate Recovery

Q: What is Medicaid Estate Recovery?

A: When a Medicaid recipient dies, the state has an enforceable debt against the recipient's estate. However, in the state of Florida, the homestead of a Medicaid recipient is a protected asset even upon the recipient's death so long as the home continues as a homestead. Assets other than the home may be protected by utilizing a trust, instead of a will, to pass the assets onto the Medicaid recipient's loved ones.

Example: Jim Smith owned two condominiums when he was qualified for Medicaid. His homestead condominium was exempt as Florida Homestead, and his second condominium was exempt because it was listed for sale when Jim applied for Medicaid. Upon his death, the state of Florida filed a lien against both condominiums. The lien on the homestead property was released because the condominium went to Jim's natural heirs under his will. However, the state was allowed to recover the cost paid to Jim by Medicaid against the non-homestead condominium because the second condominium was not exempt property.

Withdrawal From Medicaid

Q: Can I withdraw from Medicaid after qualifying for and receiving Medicaid Benefits?

A: Yes, a Medicaid recipient can withdraw from the Medicaid program by notifying the Medicaid office in writing of their desire to withdraw from receiving Medicaid benefits.

POSTSCRIPT

President Bush signed the Deficit Reduction Act of 2005 on February 8, 2006. This new federal law, which has not yet taken effect in Florida, as of the publication of this book, contains significant changes, which will eventually impact Florida Medicaid. As a practical matter, the new law contains two significant changes, as far as Florida Medicaid planning is concerned.

First, the new law changes the gifting look back period from three years, to five years. More importantly, the new law allows all gifts in the five years prior to a Medicaid application to be deemed to have occurred on the date of the Medicaid application, not the actual date of the gift. The new change in gifting rules will increase the amount of documentation required for Medicaid applications. Additionally, the new law will likely slow the processing of Medicaid applications, and significantly increase the number of Medicaid applications being denied. Accordingly, there will likely be an increased need for Medicaid applicants to seek legal assistance in obtaining Medicaid qualification.

The second major area to be impacted by the new law relates to certain annuities, which are used to obtain Medicaid qualification. A Medicaid qualifying "balloon" style single premium immediate annuity is currently a very popular strategy for obtaining Medicaid qualification for an unmarried person in Florida. The new law no longer allows the use of a "balloon" style annuity to obtain Medicaid qualification. Additionally, under the new law, if an annuity is used to obtain Medicaid qualification, the State of Florida will be named the primary beneficiary of the annuity, to reimburse the state for the Medicaid benefits paid to the Medicaid recipient. The good news is that many of the strategies currently used in Florida to obtain immediate Medicaid qualification are still available. Those strategies include, but are not limited to, the following existing strategies: personal services contracts, spousal refusal, level payout single premium immediate annuities, federally authorized trusts for the disabled and elderly individuals applying for Medicaid, as well as several other planning strategies.

A final note on this new law is that the House and the Senate passed slightly different versions of the new law. Accordingly, the issue has already been raised that the Deficit Reduction Act of 2005 may be unconstitutional on procedural grounds. Later editions of this book will contain further discussion of the Deficit Reduction Act of 2005, as the Medicaid laws change.

Chapter IV

MEDICAID QUICK REFERENCE GUIDE

3 PRONG TEST FOR MEDICAID ELIGIBILITY

1. Needs-Based Test

Generally, those that require skilled care by a nurse or nursing home on a daily basis usually will meet the needs-based standard for Medicaid eligibility. (pg.11)

2. Assets Test

Resource Allowance (Individual): $2,000 00, pg.12)
Resource Allowance (Couple): $3,000 00, (pg.13)
Min. Monthly Maintenance Needs Allowance: $1,604.00, (pg.13)
Max. Monthly Maintenance Needs Allowance: $2,489.00, (pg.14-15)
Community Spouse Resource Allowance: $99,540.00, (pg.15-16)
Monthly Personal Needs Allowance: $35.00, (pg.16)

3. Income Test

Income Cap Amount: $1,809.00, (pg.17-18)
Shelter Standard: $482.00, (pg.18-19)
Qualified Income Trust (pg.28)

Additional Considerations

Look-Back Periods (pg.24)
Divestment Penalty Divisor (pg.26)
Qualified Special Needs Trust (pg.27)
Personal Service Contract (pg.29)
Medicaid Qualifying Annuity (pg.30)
Protection of Homestead (pg.33)